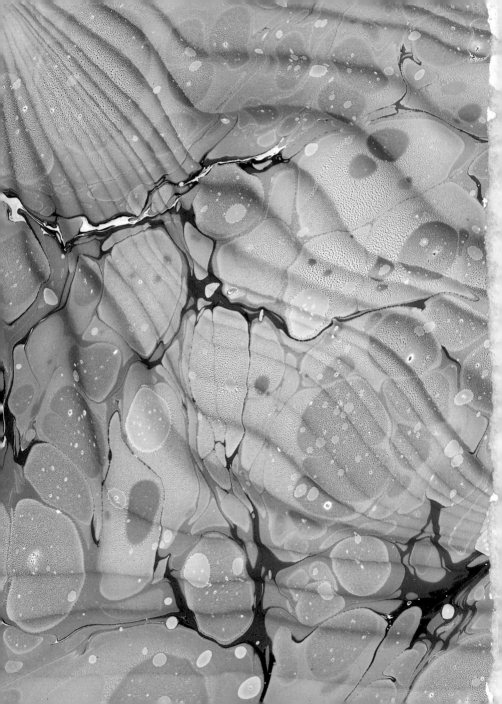

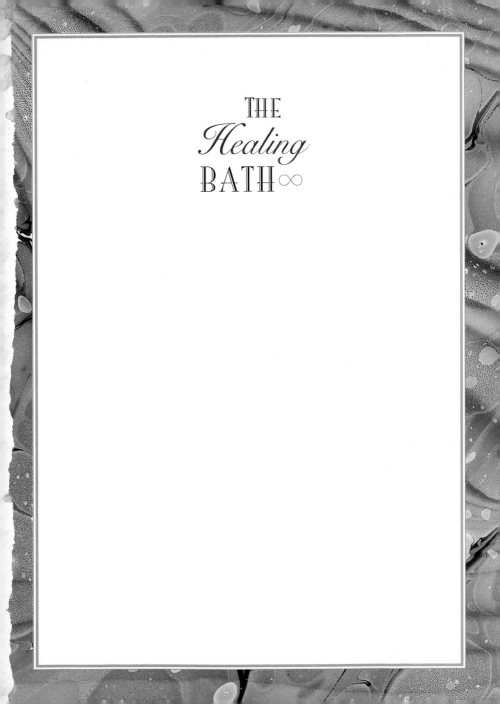

# THE *Healing* BATH ∞

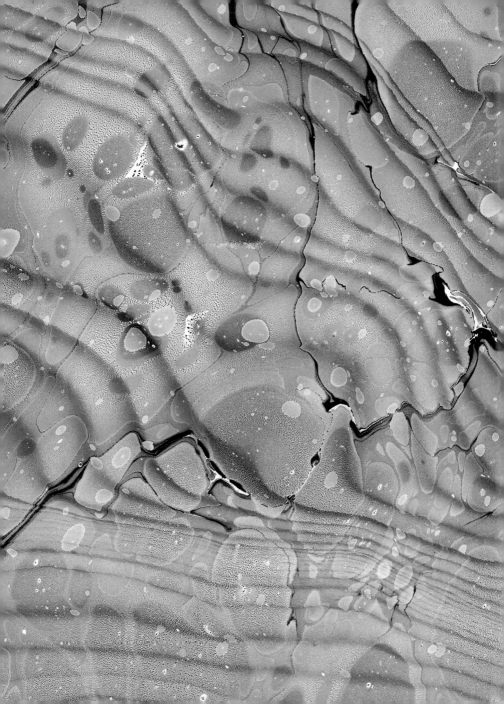

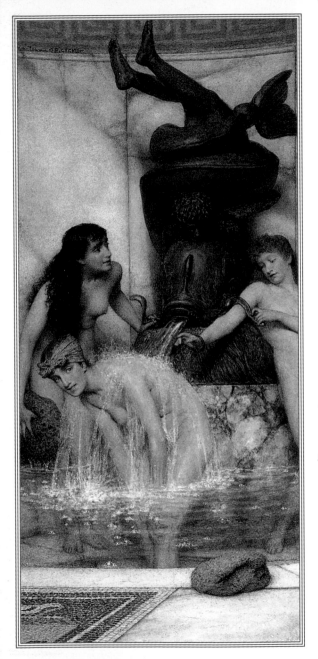

# THE *Healing* BATH ∞

*Holistic Bubbles & Soothing Soaks*

BY

## MARIBETH RIGGS

PAINTINGS BY

### SIR LAWRENCE ALMA-TADEMA

MARBLED PAPER BY

WENDY ADDISON

PENGUIN
STUDIO

PLEASE NOTE: *This book contains recipes using dried herbs, essential oils, and other ingredients that, when mixed properly and used externally, are perfectly safe. Certain of the contents, however, may cause an allergic reaction in some individuals, so reasonable care in the preparation and use of these baths is advised.*

## PENGUIN STUDIO

Published by the Penguin Group

Penguin Books USA Inc., 375 Hudson Street,
New York, New York 10014, U. S. A.

Penguin Books Ltd, 27 Wrights Lane, London W8 5TZ, England

Penguin Books Australia Ltd, Ringwood, Victoria, Australia

Penguin Books Canada Ltd, 10 Alcorn Avenue, Suite 300, Toronto, Ontario, Canada M4V 3B2

Penguin Books [N.Z] Ltd, 182–190 Wairau Road, Auckland 10, New Zealand

Penguin Books Ltd, Registered Offices: Harmondsworth, Middlesex, England

First published in 1996 by Viking Penguin, a division of Penguin Books USA Inc.

1    3    5    7    9    10    8    6    4    2

CIP Data Available

ISBN 0-670-85924-9

PRINTED IN SINGAPORE

FLY
PRODUCTIONS

# CONTENTS

∞

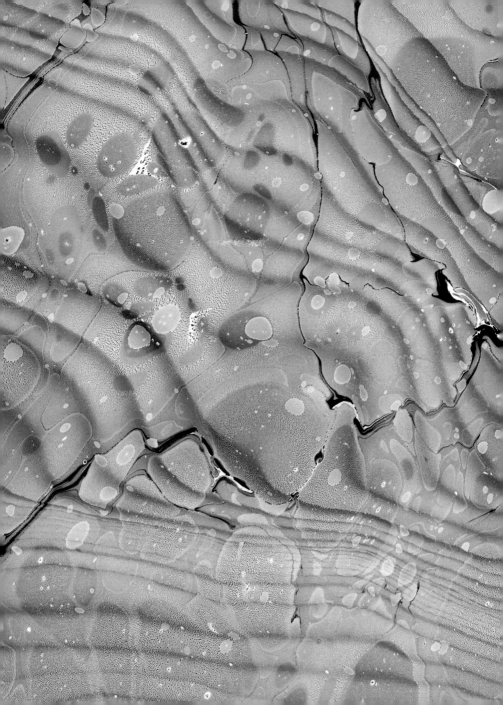

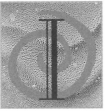

# ntroduction

*The way to health is to take an
aromatic bath and scented massage every day.*

—Hippocrates

*The Healing Bath* presents a broad spectrum of aromatherapeutic baths developed to nourish, purify, energize, or relax the body and the mind. Bathing in water enriched with concentrated infusions of botanicals and synergistic blends of essential oils is preventive health care at its most pleasurable. The marvel of these aromaceutical bath treatments is their holistic healing action. A twenty-minute soak cleanses, moisturizes, and tones the skin, simultaneously penetrating the pores to balance and fortify the respiratory, circulatory, and lymphatic systems. Inhaling the powerful scents sends fragrant signals to the olfactory bulb located in the nose. This bundle of nerves is the only place in the body where the brain is exposed. The healing aromas virtually touch the emotions, lighting the area of the brain that controls memory, intuition, relaxation, and inspiration. All aspects of being and well-being — emotional, intellectual, spiritual, and physical — are awakened and strengthened by breathing the aromas of these pure plant extracts.

Each healing bath is a stand-alone experience. The ingredients, preparation instructions, and technical tips are given separately (and sometimes repetitively for convenience) within the individual recipes. Simple directions for making bath bags, bath teas, bath salts, bath gels and bubble bath are restated as required. *The Healing Bath* offers a therapeutic bath for all seasons and all reasons: the Deep Sleep Soak for

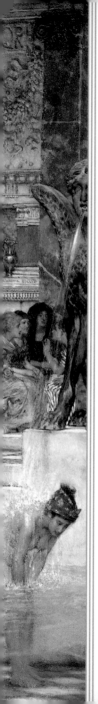

insomnia, Aromasol Vapor Cure for congestion, the Monthly FlowerBud Therapy for PMS, Morning-After Rejuvenator for hangovers, the Inspiration Solution for sparking creativity, the Skin-Silk Bath Tea for a plenitude of moisture, the Tide Pool Vitabath for detoxification, the Lovetime Elixir for sensuality, the Fresh-Up/Pep-Up for whole body rejuvenation, and the list goes on. Once you've experienced the marvelous effects of aromatherapeutic bathing, it becomes a happy habit for life.

Whether you're preparing the tranquil Tranquility Balm, the muscle-melting BathAway BackAche, the brain-tingling Jasmine Beta Boost, or the carry-on bath-in-a-bag, Jet Lag Spa To-Go, some general tips and caveats apply. Assign a separate dropper to each bottle of essential oil, or keep a container of alcohol handy for cleaning the glass dropper between applications, to avoid tainting the essences. Deliver the oils into the bath in the prescribed order to preserve the integrity and aroma of the synergistic blends. Unless specifically stated, do not apply the bath solution to your face. Essential oils, even highly diluted in a bathtub of water, are volatile and not recommended for delicate facial skin. Eye contact should be avoided, too. If you're pregnant, prepare the bath recipes at half strength and do not bathe in basil, clove, cinnamon, juniper, marjoram, myrrh, sage, thyme, peppermint, or rosemary. Pregnant women need not feel deprived. The Second Trimester Float is a glorious soak just for you (also enjoyable without a biscuit in the oven). The bath is so delightful, you'll probably continue the therapy long after the blessed event arrives.

The temperature of the bath water plays an important role in the healing treatments. The ideal water temperature for most of the baths, 95°F to 100°F, matches the body's natural temperature. Very hot water, 100°F to 104°F, opens the pores and encourages a detoxifying sweat, stimulates the lymph system, and relaxes muscle spasms. Hot baths should be brief and always followed by a cool shower to restore natural body temperature and close the pores. Cool baths, 90°F to 95°F, are recommended during pregnancy and make excellent recovery baths for convalescents. Generally speaking, bathing is drying. After every bath, a generous layer of moisturizer, applied from head to toe, is a must.

By now, you realize that essential oils are powerful healing agents and not just heavenly scents. To get the maximum results from *The Healing Bath* recipes, you need authentic aromatherapeutic products. Aromatherapy oils are stronger, purer, and more effective than perfume oils, but sometimes harder to find. The Aromatherapy Home-Shopping Network on pages 52–53 is a mail-order source guide, listing stores and catalogs where the essential oils, dried herbs, bath and skincare supplies used in the book are available.

Now it's your time for self care — close the door, turn on the tap, and take *The Healing Bath* plunge — to say thank you, Me.

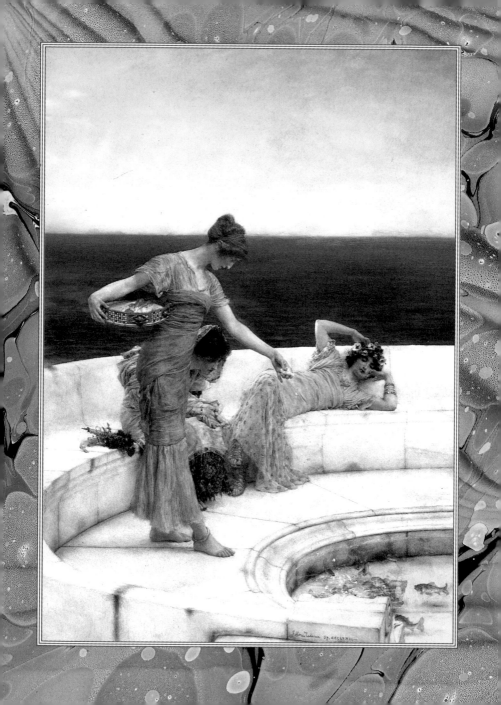

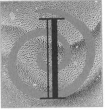

# nspiration Solution

*The debt we owe to the play of imagination*
*is incalculable.*
— Carl Gustav Jung

Feeling good about yourself is good for you. The Inspiration Solution's uplifting aroma charges your senses with a sense of optimism. The fresh fragrance of this citrus-scented soak inspires contentment, sharpens concentration, and promotes creativity. When you feel gratified and self-satisfied, good ideas just seem to flow.

## The Botanicals

*Ten Drops of Bergamot Oil*
*Eight Drops of Lemon Balm Oil*
*Eight Drops of Bay Oil*
*Five Drops of Grapefruit Oil*

The essential oils in the Inspiration Solution encourage creativity by exciting and stimulating the right side of your brain. The complex citrus formula is a bracing blend of bergamot, lemon balm, and grapefruit tempered smooth by the serene scent of bay. Breathe in these mood-elevating aromas and feel your spirits lift. Bergamot, lemon balm, bay, and grapefruit share several therapeutic applications. Their revitalizing and energizing properties are used in the treatment of depression, anxiety, stress, and fatigue. In harmony, the combined effect of these dynamically teamed essential oils is positively inspiring.

❀　❀　❀

Run your bath to a comfortable temperature, between 95°F and 100°F. When the tub is almost full, add the bergamot, the lemon balm, the bay, and the grapefruit. Deliver the oils into the bath in the prescribed order. The light, delicate oil of grapefruit is added last, to maintain its integrity against the peppery scent of bergamot. To avoid tainting your essential oils, clean your dropper with alcohol between applications, or assign each oil its own dropper. Agitate the bath water with your hand to disperse and combine the ingredients.

Sit back in the tub and get comfortable. Close your eyes, open your mouth as wide as you can, and make yourself yawn. Yoga-yawning releases tension and gives your lower facial muscles a good, toning stretch. Inhale deeply through your nose. Play a game of concentration. Try to separate the lemon-scented layers. See if your nose knows each subtle shade of citrus: spicy bergamot, clean lemon balm, warm grapefruit, and sweet bay. Feel a sense of happiness wash over you. Loll in the rejuvenating lake of inspiration until it's cool. Towel-dry vigorously. You're ready to greet the challenge of a new day with a song in your heart.

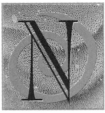utribath

*Serious illness doesn't bother me for long*
*because I am too inhospitable a host.*
— Albert Schweitzer

With the curtain rising on the 21st century, we're seeing the future foreshadowed in the present. Our children will view cellular phones and cell-level viruses as quaint benchmarks in a high-tech lifestyle we can hardly predict. Ironically, as we take our baby steps along the information highway, a renewed appreciation for the efficacy of time-honored herbal therapies is being rediscovered. The Nutribath is rich in treatment-oriented botanicals to resuscitate your system and speed recovery after a lingering New-Age flu.

## The Botanicals
*One Cup of Colloidal Oatmeal*
*Three Cups of Whole Milk*
*One Cup of Orange Flower Water*
*Five Drops of Sage Oil*
*Ten Drops of Chamomile Oil*
*Ten Drops of Orange Blossom Oil*

The Nutribath is the bath of choice for convalescents. The nourishing water feeds vital nutrients to a depleted system. B-complex vitamins suspended in a milk emollient, and water-soluble minerals — calcium and magnesium — in colloidal oatmeal, restore stamina and the skin's natural PH balance. Vitamin A and some additional calcium contained in orange blossom oil lift your spirits and counteract post-flu depression. The soothing action of sensitive chamomile oil alleviates stress, and the antiseptic properties of sage oil cleanses and freshens, inside and out.

❖　❖　❖

Run your bath to a warm temperature, between 90°F and 95°F. After an illness, the skin is super-sensitive to extremes. Slowly pour the colloidal oatmeal into the bath water, near the tap, to allow the moving water to disperse the powder. Add the whole milk. Swirl the water to combine completely. When the bath is nearly full, add the orange flower water, the sage oil, chamomile oil, and the oil of orange blossom. Agitate the water well to integrate the ingredients. The delicate, healing aroma, set off by a spring breeze of orange blossom, is grounded and welcoming.

Lie back and relax. Enjoy the sensation of the silky water washing away the staleness of prolonged bed rest. The blend of scents is pleasantly distinctive, exactly the right intensity for a weakened system or a just-well stomach. Soak for twenty minutes or longer, but at the first sign of lightheadedness leave the bath — you've had enough. Emerge from the Nutribath feeling refreshed and restored. Gently pat your sensitive skin dry, bundle in your warmest bathrobe, and get back into bed. It's never wise to push yourself.

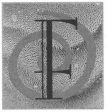

# resh-Up/Pep-Up

*Don't fight forces;*
*use them.*
— Buckminster Fuller

Retreat to rejuvenate. An atmosphere of peace and comfort are key to restoring your natural stamina. Instead of a shower that intensifies nervous energy, time out in a tub spiked with stimulating essential oils reinvigorates your senses and refreshes your body. A twist of ginger, a sparkle of cypress, a splash of ambergris, and your bath experience is a peppy perk to revive at the end of the day.

## The Botanicals

*Eight Drops of Ginger Oil*
*Ten Drops of Cypress Oil*
*Ten Drops of Ambergris Oil*

The wake-up blend of ginger, cypress, and ambergris creates a penetrating fragrance to sharpen your senses, focus your attention, and gather your forces for whatever lies ahead. The bracing solution turns the bath water into a super-cleansing and toning skin preparation, loofah-perfect for sloughing your body to baby softness. Spicy ginger stimulates circulation, raises your body temperature, and makes your skin tingle with warmth. The deep green leaves of the majestic cypress tree are the source of essential cypress oil. The dry, resinous scent reduces stress and renews your sense of balance and harmony. The smoky aroma of ambergris is comforting and familiar. Although it's not

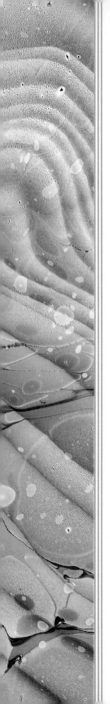

used in traditional aromatherapy, ambergris' fragrance acts to rejuvenate.

❀   ❀   ❀

The Fresh-Up/Pep-Up gives optimum results in bath water that's a bit cooler than usual, about 90°F. The temperature is perfect when you can't feel the difference between the room temperature and the water temperature. Shivering is not prescribed. The tepid temp enhances the energizing effect of the therapeutic oils. When the tub is nearly full, take a little sniff of each oil to choose your preference for the blend's dominant scent and deliver that one into the water last. The invigorating synergy of the oils is not altered, but the overall aroma is spicy by adding ginger last, serene with a cypress finish, or sweet and smoky with a final touch of ambergris. Swirl the bath water to disperse the essences thoroughly.

Place your loofah within easy reach and sink into the water. Soak for ten minutes to soften your skin before you begin your whole-body exfoliation. Start with the soles of your feet (yes, the soles), then ankles, legs, knees, and thighs, brushing upward toward your heart. Keep moistening the loofah. Use a circular motion on your stomach and chest. As you slough away the dead cells you're bringing blood to the skin's surface and stimulating your lymph system to eliminate toxins. Lie back, take a deep breath, relax, and relish your skin's rosy glow.

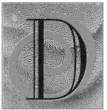

# eep Sleep Soak

*Dreams are the guardians of sleep*
*and not its disturbers.*
— Sigmund Freud

Do you retire reluctantly and then resent your alarm clock? Do your thoughts start to spin as soon as your eyes close? Nothing is more upsetting than being deprived of a full night's z-z-z. Don't panic, soak in bath water treated with sleep-inducing herbs and fragrant essential oils to bathe away insomnia and say bye-bye to sleepless nights.

## The Botanicals

*One-Half Ounce of Dried Basil*
*One-Half Ounce of Dried Sage*
*One-Quarter Ounce of Dried Marjoram*
*One-Half Ounce of Star Anise*
*Ten Drops of Clary Sage Oil*
*Ten Drops of Lavender Oil*

The botanicals in the Deep Sleep Soak combine beautifully to promote whole-body relaxation. The fragrant blend of essential oils smells wonderful and is an effective healer. Inhale the evergreen aroma of basil to banish nervous stress, tension headaches, and mental fatigue. Breathe the deep-forest scent of sage in combination with its favored partner, sweet and spicy marjoram, to warm and relax. Both soothe tired muscles and calm frayed nerves. The dreamy, licorice scent of star anise perfumes the herbaceous brew with a balancing

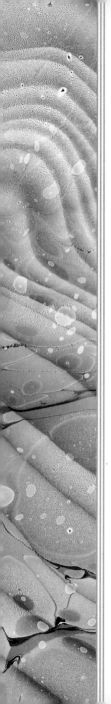

bottom note. And key to this soporific soak are the powerful sedatives, clary sage and lavender, time-honored remedies for insomnia.

❅   ❅   ❅

*To Prepare The Deep Sleep Bath Brew:* In a large, heavy-bottomed pot with a tightly fitting lid, combine the basil, sage, marjoram, star anise, and two quarts of water. Stir before heating. Bring to a boil. Lower the heat and uncover the pot to slow the boil to a simmer. Cover and continue to simmer for five minutes. Turn off the heat and steep for fifteen minutes. Strain the brew through a fine-gauge sieve into a glass pitcher. Discard the spent herbs. The infusion is dark, forest green with an overriding fragrance of languorous star anise.

Run your bath to a comfortable temperature, between 95°F and 100°F. Pour the herbal brew into the tub, near the tap, to allow the moving water to disperse the infusion. When the tub is nearly full, add the essential oils of clary sage and lavender. Swirl the bath water frequently to blend all the ingredients thoroughly.

Lower yourself into the bath. Close your eyes. This is your time. Take it — just float and relax. Feel the Deep Sleep Soak work its magic. Don't soap or scrub your skin. Soak for twenty minutes or longer, until the water is cool. Don your coziest nightclothes and tuck yourself in. Nighty-Night.

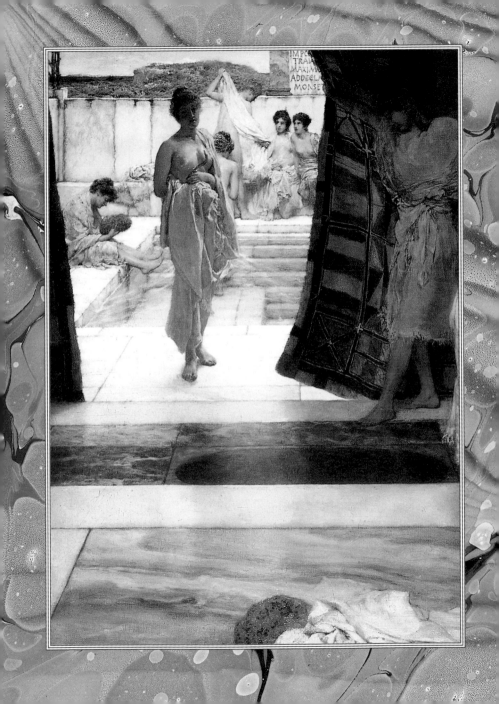

# 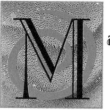ale Pamper Plunge

*Man's main task in life*
*is to give birth to himself.*
— Erich Fromm

Bathing for pleasure was once a male-only pastime. Gentlemen of leisure pampered themselves in Turkish baths and indulged in intricate, *après*-steamroom *toilettes* at exclusive men's clubs. Nowadays, labors of beauty and rejuvenation are entertained by both sexes. Prepare the Male Pamper Plunge at home (just like an aromatherapy treatment given at a state-of-the-art retreat) — an Oktoberfest bath bag, packed to bursting with bay leaves and juniper berries, afloat in spice-spiked bath water — to nurture and please the man in your life.

## The Botanicals

*One-Half Cup of Almond Meal*
*Ten Drops of Patchouli Oil*
*Fifteen Drops of Pine Balsam Oil*
*Four Drops of Juniper Oil*
*One-Half Ounce of Bay Leaves, Shredded*
*One-Half Ounce of Juniper Berries, Crushed*
*Terry Washcloth*
*One-Half Yard of Cotton String*
*Fifteen Drops of Amber Oil*
*Eight Drops of Musk Oil*

The bracing aroma of the Male Pamper Plunge combines herbs and oils distilled from the bark, tree resin, new leaves, and ripe berries of fragrant forest plants especially appealing to men. An Oktoberfest bath bag filled with silken grains of almond meal tossed fragrant with a bouquet of smoky, sensual patchouli, spirited pine balsam, stimulating bay, and pleasantly pungent juniper treats the emotions and tones the skin. The lightly astringent bath water, redolent with the allure of musk and amber, lingers all day.

❊　　❊　　❊

*To Prepare The Oktoberfest Bath Bag:* In a glass bowl, combine the almond meal, patchouli oil, pine balsam oil, and juniper oil. Stir with a spoon or mix by hand thoroughly to blend the oils with the almond meal. The grainy texture of the almond meal is barely affected by the addition of the oils. Mix in the shredded bay leaves and the crushed juniper berries. Toss and stir to distribute the ingredients evenly and completely.

Open the washcloth and lay it on a flat surface. Mound the mixture in the center of the washcloth. Raise the corners of the washcloth and twist them closed to form a tightly packed bundle. Wind the cotton string around the top, four or five times, until almost all the string is used. Finish with a tight knot to close the bath bag securely.

Run the bath to a comfortable temperature, between 95°F and 100°F. When the tub is almost full, launch the bath bag. Give it a squeeze to release a silky stream of forest-scented

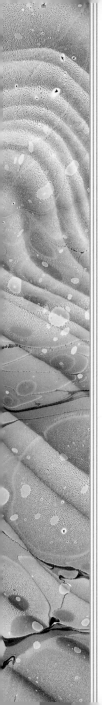

almond meal into the bath water. Add the amber oil and the musk oil. Agitate the water to disperse the oils evenly.

Immerse quickly in the goose-bump warm water. This is pure sensual pleasure. Float away to a fantasy forest of pungent juniper trees, pine-covered trails, and ripe running sap. Rub the bath bag over the body to condition and slough away dry, rough skin. The prickly-soft terrycloth stimulates circulation and makes the skin tingle. Your male "guinea pig" exits his watery cocoon feeling fresh, happy, and grateful.

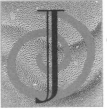

# Jet Lag Spa To-Go

*Man unites himself with the world
in the process of creation.*
— Erich Fromm

Even the most experienced travelers suffer from the dread condition known as jet lag. Traveling at six hundred miles per hour in a pressurized, temperature-controlled cabin, not to mention the hours spent in a cramped seat, definitely takes its toll on your body and your psyche. The Jet Lag Spa To-Go is portable aromatherapeutical relief to the rescue. A twenty-minute layover in the healing spa bath resets your inner clock to the correct time zone. So, pack up your aromas in your new cosmetics' bag and smile.

## The Carry-On Spa Kit

*Twelve Drops of Rosemary Oil*

*Ten Drops of Lemongrass Oil*

*Eight Drops of Geranium Oil*

*Four Drops of Peppermint Oil*

*Four Drops of Juniper Oil*

*One-Quarter Ounce Amber Glass Bottle with Screw-Top*

*Glass Dropper*

*Travel-Size Bar of Peppermint Soap*

*Travel-Size Atomizer of Mineral Water*

*Black-Out Eye Shade*

*Ear Plugs*

No matter what time it is when you touch down, the Jet Lag Spa makes it the right time. The clean and clear combination of fresh rosemary, sweet lemongrass, spicy geranium, peppy peppermint, and pungent juniper soaks away stress, calms nerves, settles your stomach, decongests your sinuses, soothes sore body parts, refreshes your skin, shortens recovery time, and lifts your flagging spirits. The reviving and relaxing blend of essential oils in the Jet Lag Spa does all of that. And the scent is sensational!

❈   ❈   ❈

*To Prepare The Carry-On Spa Kit:* Into the quarter-ounce amber glass bottle, drop the oils of rosemary, lemongrass, geranium, peppermint, and juniper. Screw the lid on tight. Agitate well, but gently, to combine the oils. Into a small zippered bag with compartments, pack the bottle of bath oil, the glass dropper, the travel-size bar of peppermint soap, the travel-size spray can of mineral water, the black-out eye shade, and the ear plugs.

*Upon Arrival:* Call room service. Order a bottle of still mineral water, a bucket of ice, and a side order of sliced lemon for a refreshing beverage to sip while you soak. Run your bath to a comfortable temperature, not too hot or you'll become even more dehydrated. When the tub is nearly full, empty the bottle of pre-blended oils into the bath water. Swirl the water gently with your hand to combine evenly. Lower the window shade, close the curtains, and turn off the light. Slide into the inviting bath. Slip on the eye shade and put in the ear plugs.

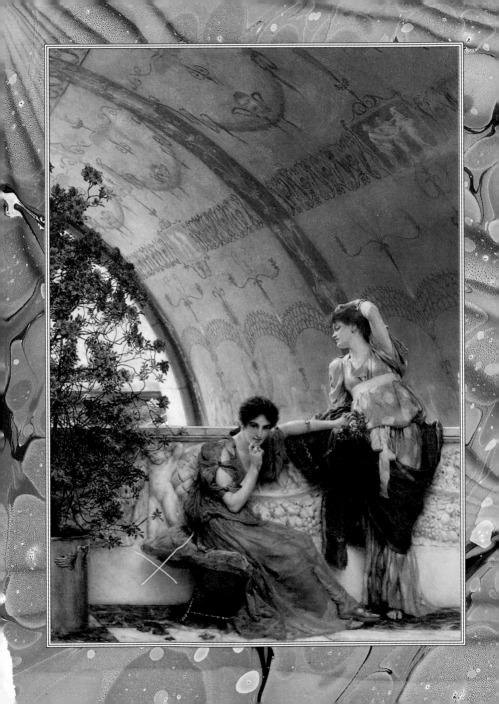

Lay back in sightless, soundless, watery space. Inhale the restorative aromas. Ten to fifteen minutes in timeless, near-weightless isolation feels like eternity. Remove the eye shade and the ear plugs and return to realtime, refreshed and revived. Lather all over with tingling, creamy peppermint soap. Mist your face with a rehydrating spray of mineral water.

Towel off, apply a generous layer of moisturizer to satisfy your mighty thirsty skin, and turn on the tube to see what's going on in the world. You're ready.

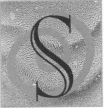

# Spicy Rose Relaxercise

*A sound mind in a sound body is a short but full*
*description of a happy state in this world.*
— John Locke

The prescribed (and preferred) after-exercise activity is a relaxing bath in hot water. The Spicy Rose Relaxercise is a water workout to cool down your muscles, condition your skin, and center your mind. Float the sweet and spicy Your-Time bath bag in the rich, rose-velvet bath water to extend the physical and mental benefits of your calorie burn.

## The Botanicals

*One-and-One-Half Ounces of Powdered Orris Root*

*Fifteen Drops of Vanilla Oil*

*Four Drops of Cinnamon Oil*

*Four Drops of Clove Oil*

*One Tablespoon of Sweet Almond Oil*

*One Vanilla Bean Pod, Finely Chopped*

*Ten Whole Cloves, Crushed*

*One Cinnamon Stick, Crushed*

*Terry Washcloth*

*One-Half Yard of Cotton String*

*Ten Drops of Rose Geranium Oil*

*Fifteen Drops of Rose Oil*

Exquisite rose, the goddess of mood-altering florals, uplifts, increases self-confidence, relieves stress, and makes you feel and smell

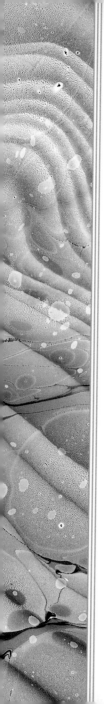

beautiful. The rose geranium back enhances the rose aroma tenfold. Squeeze the Your-Time bath bag, filled to the brim with intoxicating scents, and deliver a satin ribbon of sweetness into the rose-rich waterbed. Warming vanilla, rousing clove, sexy cinnamon, deepen the faux-violet scent of powdered orris root, transforming the bath water to soft silk.

❊    ❊    ❊

*To Prepare The Your-Time Bath Bag:* In a glass bowl combine the powdered orris root, the vanilla oil, the cinnamon oil, the clove oil, and the sweet almond oil. Stir with a spoon or mix by hand to combine the oils with the powdered orris root thoroughly. The soft texture of the powdered orris root is made lightly moist by the addition of the oils. Mix in the finely chopped vanilla bean, the crushed cloves, and the crushed cinnamon stick. Toss and stir to distribute the ingredients evenly and completely.

Open the washcloth and lay it on a flat surface. Mound the mixture in the center of the washcloth. Raise the corners and twist them closed to form a tightly packed bundle. Wind the cotton string around the top, four or five times, until almost all the string is used. Finish with a tight knot to seal the bag securely.

Run your bath to a comfortable temperature, between 95° and 100°F. When the bath is nearly full, set the bath bag afloat. Squeeze it to release an opalescent trail of heaven-scent powder into the water. Add the oil of rose geranium and the oil of rose. Swish the cream-soft bath water with your hand to distribute the oils evenly. Deliver the oils into the bath in the prescribed order to allow the scent of "true" rose to shine.

Plant yourself in the floating rose garden. Shivers of ecstasy and waves of happiness wash over you. Gently rub your body with the highly spiced bath bag. The penetrating perfume smells indescribably wonderful. The aroma is undeniably euphoric. Languish in luxury until the water is cool. Before you dress, mist from head to toe with rosewater. You'll sport a rose silk suit all day.

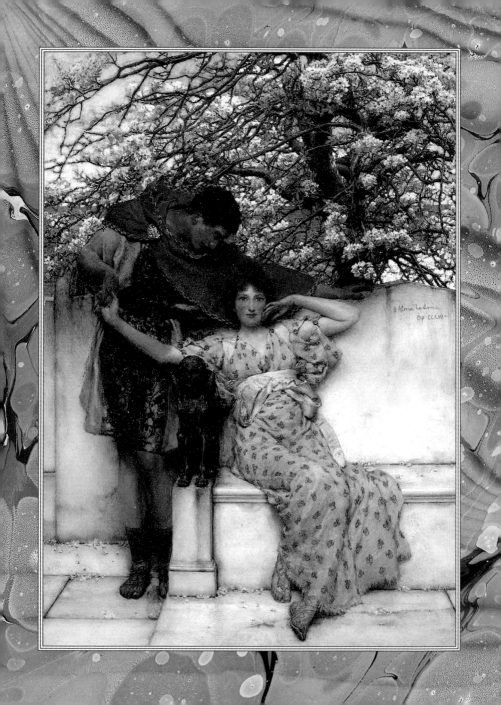

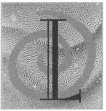# ovetime Elixir

*The meeting of two personalities is like the contact*
*of two chemical substances: if there is any reaction,*
*both are transformed.*— Carl Gustav Jung

The Lovetime Elixir is an aromadesiac, a blend of exotic essential oils that inspire sensuality and enhance sexual vitality. Wrap your body in this cloak of seductive scents to stimulate desire and shake off inhibitions. The potent combination of aromatic essences, tender cardamom, suggestive ylang ylang, intimate patchouli, are a sultan's gift gathered from the trees and flowers growing in the love-palace gardens. Bathe in the warm, sensuous water to heighten the elixir's arousing affect and make you feel sexy from head to toe.

## The Botanicals

*Fifteen Drops of Cardamom Oil*
*Eight Drops of Ylang Ylang Oil*
*Ten Drops of Patchouli Oil*

The Lovetime Elixir lights the flame of love. The melting warmth of infatuating cardamom, the bewitching fragrance of beguiling ylang ylang, and the profound aroma of romantic patchouli ignites desire to put you (and your partner) in the mood for love. Cardamom, the initiator, boosts self-confidence. Ylang ylang, the temptress, sheds inhibitions. Patchouli, the persistent, stimulates sexual energy. With synergistic zest this endless-love potion attracts love to realize love.

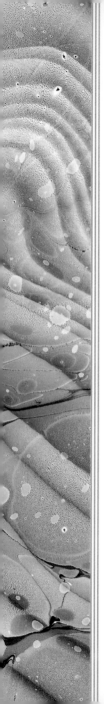

❆    ❆    ❆

As night falls, on a day when lovemaking seems likely, indulge in a candlelit Lovetime Elixir bath. Decorate your bathroom with clusters of tall white candles, strategically placed around the room.

Run your bath to a comfortable temperature, between 95°F and 100°F. When the tub is nearly full, add the oil of cardamom, the oil of ylang ylang, and the oil of patchouli. Agitate the water to combine the oils completely. The essences bond perfectly to simulate the scented integrity of a precious Oriental perfume.

Light the candles and relax into the steaming bath water. Don't soap or scrub your skin, surrender to your senses. The Lovetime Elixir is an olfactory turn-on. Inhale the heady scents to feel sexy all over. Languish in the voluptuously scented bath water. As the candles flicker and glow, fantasize . . . once upon a romantic time, long, long ago, a love-struck young man (in tights) delighted a lovely young woman with a sweet-smelling flower and courtly love was born.

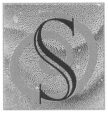

# Skin-Silk Bath Tea

*Our skin, as on a screen, the gamut of life's experiences*
*is projected: emotions surge, sorrows penetrate, and*
*beauty finds its depth.* — A. Montagu

Serve rehydrating Skin-Silk Bath Tea to quench your skin's thirst for moisture. The replenishing blend of aromatic botanicals penetrates the pores to nourish, sooth, and saturate. The therapeutic properties of the radiantly fragrant herbs and essential oils are absorbed directly into your body to reward your senses and restore moisture to your skin.

## The Botanicals

*One Ounce of Slippery Elm Powder*
*One-Half Cup of Honey*
*One-and-One-Half Ounces of Dried Deer Tongue, Shredded*
*Three Cups of Whole Milk*
*Eight Drops of Ylang Ylang*
*Ten Drops of Sandalwood Oil*

The Skin-Silk Bath Tea is a thoroughly holistic soak. The soothing emollient slippery elm powder, the dewy humectant honey, and the gentle cleanser whole milk suspend the nutritive essential oils in absorbent sweet-cream moisture. The grassy, mock-vanilla scent of deer tongue adds green focus to fertile, flowery ylang ylang and warm, spicy sandalwood. Ylang ylang and sandalwood, the yin and yang of essential oils, work together in perfect harmony to heal, soothe, and rejuvenate.

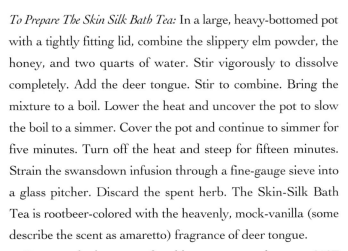

*To Prepare The Skin Silk Bath Tea:* In a large, heavy-bottomed pot with a tightly fitting lid, combine the slippery elm powder, the honey, and two quarts of water. Stir vigorously to dissolve completely. Add the deer tongue. Stir to combine. Bring the mixture to a boil. Lower the heat and uncover the pot to slow the boil to a simmer. Cover the pot and continue to simmer for five minutes. Turn off the heat and steep for fifteen minutes. Strain the swansdown infusion through a fine-gauge sieve into a glass pitcher. Discard the spent herb. The Skin-Silk Bath Tea is rootbeer-colored with the heavenly, mock-vanilla (some describe the scent as amaretto) fragrance of deer tongue.

Run your bath to a comfortable temperature, between 95°F and 100°F. Pour in the bath tea, near the tap, to disperse the infusion. When the tub is half full, add the whole milk. Agitate the water to combine. Just before you turn off the faucet, add the ylang ylang and the sandalwood. Swirl to combine the oils with the *café au lait* bath water.

Tie up your hair and immerse yourself in plush velvet comfort. Luxuriate. Let the penetrating solution turn your skin to shining silk. The Skin-Silk Bath Tea is a plenitude of dewy moisture, but please don't apply it to the delicate, combination skin on your face. Essential oils, even highly diluted, are volatile. *Après le bain,* bring your face up to the level of your honey-hydrated body, moisturize with your favorite face cream. You'll be stroking-soft for days.

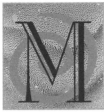

# Morning-After Rejuvenator

*I must get out of these wet clothes
and into a dry Martini.*
— Robert Benchley

The day-after the night-before is an eye-crossing, head-pounding, stomach-lurching punishment. It's not fair, even if you were naughty (on purpose). Alcohol acts as a diuretic, the dehydration that results is the main cause of the horrible hangover. Be kind to yourself the morning after, submerge and purge in the aromatherapeutic version of the hair-of-the-dog to emerge almost unscathed. A cup of peppermint tea, tubside, to sip as you soak, is recommended.

## The Botanicals

*Six Drops of Eucalyptus Oil*
*Ten Drops of Peppermint Oil*
*Six Drops of Myrrh Oil*
*Ten Drops of Sandalwood Oil*

The essential oils in the Morning-After Rejuvenator are target treatments for the parts of your body calling out for help — your head, your tummy, and your jangled nerves. Sniffing and sipping, as you're soaking in the medicinal water, delivers healing ingredients directly into your system, promoting whole body rehydration, pain relief, and renewed vigor. The memorable scent of eucalyptus is penetrating and camphor-like. Most people can identify it easily after smelling it only once. Eucalyptus is an effective anesthetic, decongestant, and astringent.

∞ *25* ∞

The clean, medicinal scent is stimulating and head-clearing. The warmth of eucalyptus is counterpoint to cooling peppermint. Also a stimulant, anesthetic, astringent, and powerful decongestant, the active ingredient in peppermint, menthol, goes to work immediately to heal your upset stomach and stop the pounding in your head. One whiff of peppermint's lively aroma makes you alert and focused. Mellow myrrh and spicy sandalwood are sweet foils to pungent eucalyptus and peppy peppermint. These two exotics give the blend its lovely perfume. Not just pretty aromas, both are astringent to eliminate toxins and effective digestives to settle a touchy tummy.

❀   ❀   ❀

Run your bath to a comfortable temperature, between 95°F and 100°F. When the bath is nearly full, add the eucalyptus, peppermint, myrrh, and sandalwood. Swirl the water gently with your hand to combine well. Deliver the essences into the bath in the prescribed order with delicately scented sandalwood the mellow, finishing touch. Remember to clean your dropper between applications to avoid tainting your bottles of oils.

Put your mug of tea within easy reach. Rest in the bath until the water cools. The soothing soak relieves the hangover symptoms almost immediately. Use the rest of the time to resolve never to overindulge again (until the next time).

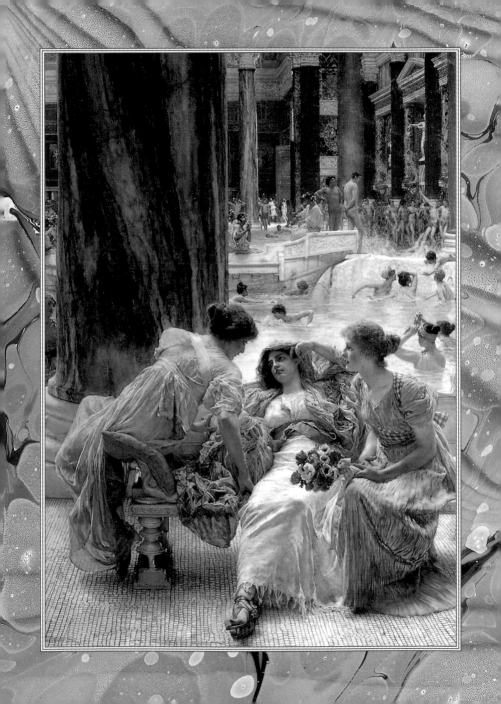

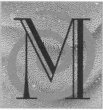

# onthly FlowerBud Therapy

*To [she] who looks upon the world rationally,*
*the world in its turn presents a rational aspect.*
— Georg Wilhelm Friedrich Hegel

Can we talk? Every woman recognizes the symptoms of Premenstrual Syndrome: Radical mood swings, junk food binges, and frenzied shopping sprees are the signposts of this quirky disorder. Whether you're an infrequent sufferer, or one of the truly unfortunate on an emotional seesaw every month, help is here. Cocooning in the PMS FlowerBud Therapy bath calms your nerves, diminishes the free-floating cloud of gloom, and takes the fretful edge off the arrival of your fair-weather "friend."

## The Botanicals

*One-Half Ounce of Dried Comfrey Root*
*One Ounce of Dried Rosebuds*
*One Ounce of Dried Lavender Flowers*
*Two Tablespoons of Dried Thyme*
*Ten Drops of Lavender Oil*
*Ten Drops of Rose Oil*
*Fifteen Drops of Jasmine Oil*

The aromaceuticals in the Monthly FlowerBud Therapy bath form a dynamic floral synergy that reduces stress and promotes whole-body relaxation. The antidepressant rose, the sedative lavender, the euphoriant jasmine, and the stimulant thyme are suspended in a decoction of the soothing emollient comfrey root. This hardworking plant accelerates and heightens the therapeutic action of the flower botanicals.

❁　❁　❁

*To Prepare The Floating Garden Tub Tea:* In a large, heavy-bottomed pot with a tightly fitting lid, combine the comfrey root, rosebuds, lavender flowers, thyme, and two quarts of water. Stir the floating garden before heating. Bring to a boil. Lower the heat and uncover to slow the boil to a simmer. Cover and continue to simmer for five minutes. Turn off the heat. Steep for fifteen minutes. Strain the decoction through a fine-gauge sieve into a glass pitcher. Discard the spent herbs. The floral liqueur is a warm caramel color with an invigorating, fiery-flower signature scent.

Run your bath to a comfortable temperature, between 95°F and 100°F. As the bath fills, pour in the tub tea near the tap to disperse evenly. When the tub is nearly full, deliver the essential oils into the water in the prescribed order. Swirl the water to incorporate the oils.

Now it's time to make yourself well. Submerge to the chin in the healing water. Until recently, doctors prescribed forbearance and bed rest to alleviate PMS, dismissing the condition as a figment of the unconscious female collective. In the time it takes to give yourself a hug (you deserve one for taking control) a great wave of relief washes over you as tense muscles unwind and anxious stress melts away. Yes, you're one smart lady.

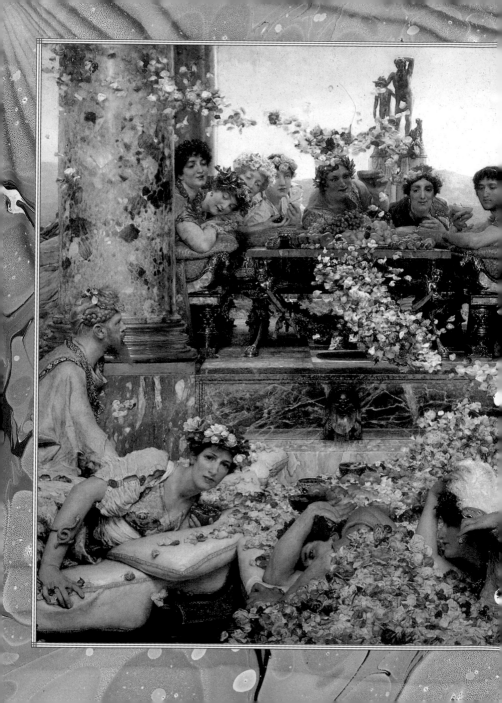

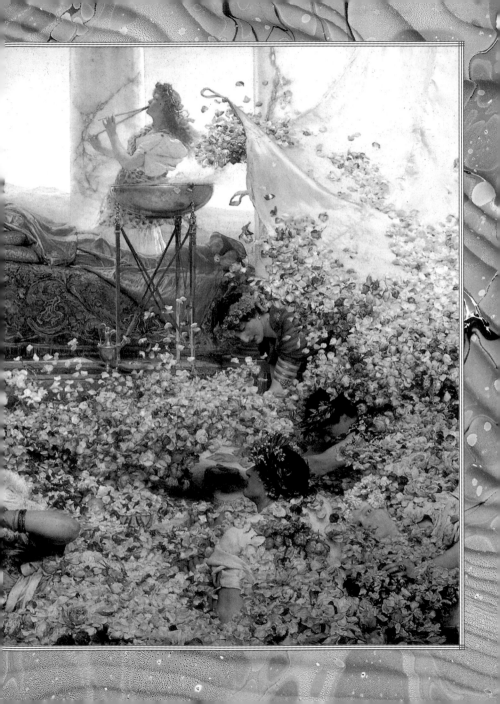

# 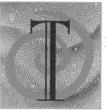ide Pool Vitabath

*To sense the ebb and flow of the tides is to
have a knowledge of things that are as nearly
eternal as any earthly life can be.* — R. Carson

A seaweed and salt soak beautifies, tones, and strengthens the skin's
natural elasticity, enhances the immune system, and reduces cellulite.
Sounds like a miracle and it practically is. Seaweed is the *botanique du
jour* among dietitians, cosmeticians, and New Age physicians. Here on the
Pacific Rim, we're almost blasé when it comes to extolling the curative
power of this ocean green, but word of seaweed's healing and cosmetic
achievements are turning up in international science journals *and* foreign
fashion magazines.

## The Botanicals

*One Ounce of Dried Kombu Seaweed*
*One Cup of Borax*
*One Tablespoon of Sea Salt*
*One Tablespoon of Powdered Cosmetic Clay*
*Twelve Drops of Spearmint Oil*
*Eight Drops of Lemongrass Oil*

Kombu, a member of the large family of "sea vegetables" known as
seaweed, is packed with vitamins, minerals, nutrients, fiber, and
phytochemicals. Bathing in an infusion of kombu nourishes the system
and hydrates the skin. The minerals and trace elements in seaweed are

akin to the chemicals found in the body's natural fluids (sweat, tears, etc.). Thus, the nutrient-rich solution is easily absorbed through the pores of the skin. Boost the efficacy of the bath water with the Rhythms Of The Sea blend of super-absorbent borax, detoxifying sea salt, soothing and softening cosmetic clay, tingling and toning spearmint oil, and refreshing oil of lemongrass to recondition your skin and regenerate your system.

❀  ❀  ❀

*To Prepare The Rhythms Of The Sea Bath Salt:* In a medium-sized bowl, combine the borax, sea salt, and cosmetic clay. Whisk to blend thoroughly. Add the spearmint oil and the lemongrass oil. Whisk until the mixture is smooth and the ingredients are well incorporated. Cover and set aside for at least one hour to allow the aromas to develop.

*To Prepare The Sea Vegetable Infusion*: In a large, heavy-bottomed pot with a tightly fitting lid, combine the kombu and two quarts of water. Stir before heating. Bring to a boil. The rehydrated kombu doubles its dehydrated size. Lower the heat and uncover the pot to slow the boil to a simmer. Cover and continue to simmer for five minutes. Turn off the heat. Steep for fifteen minutes. Strain the seaweed infusion through a mesh sieve into a glass pitcher and set aside. Discard the spent seaweed. The lovely, light-green Tide Pool solution is silky smooth and ocean scented.

Run your bath water hot, hot, as hot as you can stand it, between 98°F and 100°F plus. If you're a hot tub afficionado you've built up a tolerance to the heat, if not, be careful. (Over 95°F, you feel each additional degree as though it was an additional ten.) Don't overdo it. Pour the seaweed infusion into the bath, near the tap, to allow the turbulent water to disperse the solution. When the tub is nearly full, add the bath salts. Swirl the water with your hand to combine the ingredients well.

Now you're in for a treat. Your heated saltwater pool looks and smells like the sea with a pleasant spearmint tingle. Soak in the steaming water to induce a deep-cleansing sweat. The heat opens the skin's pores to receive the water's nourishment and release the body's toxins. After about fifteen minutes, stand up and turn on the shower. Let the hot water out of the tub while you shower in the cool water to close your pores. The drying effect of the hot water and the astringency of the sea salt solution requires lots of moisturizer all over for a finishing touch.

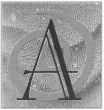# loe V. Clarifying Tonic

The reward for giving your skin first-quality care is a radiant glow. The Aloe V. Clarifying Tonic refines the texture of your skin by deep-cleansing, toning, and purifying. The moisture-gathering solution flushes impurities to leave your skin immaculate and supple. Deeply refreshing, the aromatic blend clarifies your mood, too; uplifting and serene, the combined scents smooth frown lines and relax tense facial muscles.

## The Botanicals

*One-Half Cup of Pearl Barley*
*One-Half Ounce of Dried Chamomile Flowers*
*One Cup of Aloe Vera Gel*
*Ten Drops of Grapefruit Oil*

A pore-cleansing soak in Barley & Chamomile Tub Tonic treated with Aloe & Grapefruit Clarifying Gel is pure and perfect skincare from Mother Nature's spa. Pearl barley, a mucilage, soothes skin flare-ups from pimples to psoriasis. Antiseptic chamomile reduces puffiness, nourishes new cells, and shrinks broken capillaries. The moisturizing humectant aloe vera purifies and clarifies the skin's texture. And gently astringent grapefruit oil tones and cleanses right down to the sebaceous glands to balance combination skin, fade stretch marks, and diminish cellulite.

❀ ❀ ❀

*To Prepare The Barley & Chamomile Tub Tonic:* In a large, heavy-bottomed pot with a tightly fitting lid, combine the pearl barley and two quarts of water. Bring to a boil. Lower the heat and uncover the pot to slow the boil to a simmer. Cover and simmer for twenty minutes. Add the chamomile flowers and simmer for ten minutes more. Turn off the heat and steep for fifteen minutes. Strain the infusion through a fine-gauge sieve into a glass pitcher. Discard the spent botanicals. The tub tea is daisy-au-lait with a lovely aroma of chamomile dancing in a field of earth-sweet barley.

*To Prepare The Aloe & Grapefruit Clarifying Gel:* In a small bowl, combine the aloe gel and the grapefruit oil. Whisk to blend thoroughly. The smooth gel smells deliciously uplifting.

Run your bath to a comfortable temperature, between 95°F and 100°F. Pour the tub tonic into the bath, near the tap, to disperse the infusion evenly. When the bath is half full, add the clarifying gel. Swirl the water to combine the botanicals. The bathwater is smooth and soft with a sunny-day scent.

Soak in the purifying solution without soaping or scrubbing. The softening and toning action begins within minutes. Treat your face to a facial treatment, too. Cover your face with a drenched washcloth. Leave it on for several minutes until the water cools. (After bath, splash cold water on your face to close the pores before applying moisturizer.) Remain in the tub for as long as you like. Bathe in aloe vera once a week to see a positive change in the texture of your skin.

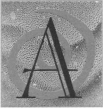# A romasol Vapor Cure

*The first wealth*
*is health.*
— Ralph Waldo Emerson

Back to basics botanically is the best relief for the stuffy, sneezy head and achy, feverish body of a cold or upper respiratory infection. There's no cure for the common cold virus, but the symptoms are treatable. The Aromasol Vapor Cure helps to drain, detoxify, and restore balance to your congested system. Taking the cure in bath form is especially effective. Breathing in the medicinal fumes decongests the respiratory system and soaking in the healing hot water penetrates the lymph system and stimulates circulation. The aromaceuticals target the afflicted areas and the steaming water sends the essences where they do the most good — straight up your nose!

## The Botanicals

*Eight Drops of Eucalyptus Oil*
*Five Drops of Wintergreen Oil*
*Five Drops of Pennyroyal Oil*
*Five Drops of Cinnamon Oil*

The intense scent and penetrating properties of eucalyptus oil are the centerpiece of this healing bath. Eucalyptus does it all: decongests, disinfects, and increases absorption of oxygen into red blood cells. Eucalyptus, in concert with the detoxifying expectorant wintergreen, the antiseptic, antiviral pennyroyal, and the stimulating astringent

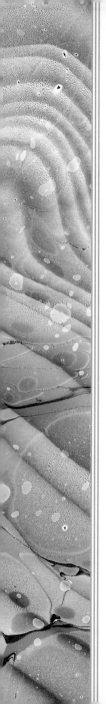

cinnamon is strong herbal medicine. Those are the physical properties. The combined psychological benefits are just as impressive and important. All four essential oils are stimulating, inspiring, and focusing to make you well mentally. The Aromasol Vapor Cure is broad spectrum relief.

❉  ❉  ❉

Run the bathwater to a steaming-hot temperature, between 98°F and 100°F plus. If your symptoms don't include fever, dizziness, or nausea, the self-induced, light sweat speeds the elimination of toxins (if they do, you shouldn't be taking a bath). When the tub is nearly full, deliver the oils into the water in the prescribed order. The triplemint blend is specially formulated to be piercing and invasive. Agitate the water to combine thoroughly. A cloud of healing aromatic steam transforms your bathroom into a vapor room.

Settle into the skin-tingling water. Inhale deeply. Hold the vapor in your lungs for a few seconds before exhaling. Let your breath out slowly and deeply. Repeat the process several times. Gently exfoliate your body with a washcloth (not your face, these oils are too volatile for prolonged contact with delicate facial skin). You don't need soap, the bath water is super-cleansing. Gently towel-dry. Apply a light layer of moisturizer. Stay warm and away from drafts. The Aromasol Vapor Cure is prescribed once a day until you're back on your feet.

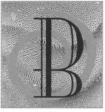# BathAway BackAche

*Anatomy is
destiny.*
— Sigmund Freud

Every day millions spend millions on over-the-counter cure-alls and patent-medicine panaceas in search of relief from lower back pain. The most common causes are lifestyle related — stress, poor posture, overweight, excessive exercise; the symptoms are chronic, striking without warning — muscle spasm, swelling, fatigue, pulsing pain; and as universal as this ailment is, controversy rages *ad nauseum* over effective treatments — heat, ice, exercise, bed rest. If you've suffered, then you've tried these (and more). Eventually, one simple therapy emerges from the many — a muscle-melting bath in hot water, doctored with aromatic thermaceuticals delivers honest relief to tense, aching muscles and stiff, swollen joints.

## The Botanicals

*One-And-One-Half Cups of Evaporated Milk*
*Eight Drops of Camphor Oil*
*Ten Drops of Cajeput Oil*

BathAway BackAche is a thermabath. The temperature of the bath water jump-starts the aromaceutical action to deep heat and heal muscles in distress. The blend of volatile oils is held in suspended combination by the evaporated milk. The soothing emulsion keeps your skin well-coated for continuous topical relief. Count on camphor and cajeput to

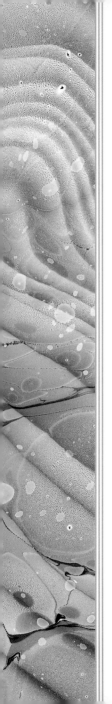

break the cycle of muscles in spasm. In synergy, camphor and cajeput are anti-inflammatory to reduce painful swelling, penetrating to stimulate circulation, and thermal to "defrost" stiff joints and muscles.

❀    ❀    ❀

Run your bath water hot, between 98°F and 100°F plus. Strong heat is tantamount to the treatment. Perch carefully on the side of the tub to prepare the water. Don't bend over to mix the ingredients (you probably can't anyway). Pour the evaporated milk into the bath, near the tap, to allow the running water to disperse the creamy substance. When the bath is nearly full add the camphor oil and the cajeput oil. Swirl the water vigorously to combine the oils thoroughly with the enriched water.

Carefully lower yourself into the tub. Take your time. Give your skin a chance to adjust to the temperature. When you can, totally immerse yourself. Breathe in the penetrating, warm-wood fragrance. Feel your muscles go limp and the pain virtually melt away. The miraculous relief is total — but temporary. The deep-heat blend may numb the pain completely, but it gradually comes back as the muscles cool to room temperature. The treatment leaves your back muscles loose and vulnerable, rest for at least an hour after bathing. BathAway once a day until your back is back to normal.

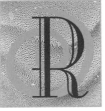

# Reflexology Foot Spa

*The human body is
the best picture of the human soul.*
— Ludwig Wittgenstein

Don't wait until your feet ache, save your soles with a simple two-step routine that pairs pampering and prevention. The path to super health is through your feet. Step one is a refreshing, fragrant footbath that lifts your spirits and your arches. Step two is a foot massage that regulates body functions, energizes your system, and makes your whole body feel great. The combination of aromatherapy and reflexology are giant steps to feeling well and staying well.

## The Botanicals:

*Four Sprigs of Fresh Rosemary*
*Two-Inch Slice of Fresh Ginger*
*Eight Drops of Rosemary Oil*
*Five Drops of Clove Oil*
*Five Drops of Lemon Verbena Oil*

Soak your tootsies in a toe-tingling tonic to stimulate circulation, relax sore soles, and refresh, tone, and moisturize the hardworking skin on your feet. The Reflexology Foot Spa is a foot saver. Alert rosemary uplifts, promotes clear thinking, and tones the skin. Active ginger stimulates, raises body temperature, and strengthens the nervous system. Aromatic clove energizes, anesthetizes, and disinfects. Dynamic

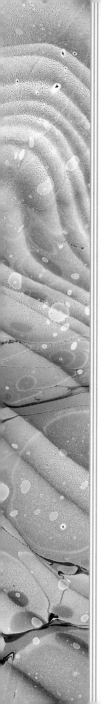

lemon verbena accelerates mental processes, focuses energy, and increases stamina. The aromatic alliance of scents inspires self-confidence and puts a bounce in your step.

❀    ❀    ❀

*To Prepare The Toning Toe Tonic:* In a large, heavy-bottomed pot with a tightly fitting lid, combine the rosemary sprigs, the slice of fresh ginger, and two quarts of water. Bring to a boil. Lower the heat and uncover the pot to slow the boil to a simmer. Cover and continue to simmer for five minutes. Turn off the heat and steep for fifteen minutes. Strain the decoction through a sieve into a glass pitcher. Discard the spent herbs. The aromatic essence is herb green with an invigorating scent of ginger, splashed licorice-cool by fragrant rosemary.

*The Foot Spa:* Sit in a straight-back chair with a rubber basin at your feet. The basin should be large enough to fit your feet side by side comfortably. Fill half way to the top with "toe tea." Add the essential oils of rosemary, clove, and lemon verbena. Swirl the water to combine completely. Place your feet in the basin. Add more tea, if necessary, to cover your ankles. Drape a bath towel over the top to trap the heat. Soak for fifteen minutes or until the water is cool. Vigorously rub your feet dry to slough away dead skin cells and stimulate circulation. Apply lots of your favorite moisturizer.

*The Reflexology Massage:* Arrange yourself comfortably on the floor or on your bed, somewhere you're able to massage the soles of your feet without bending over or assuming an

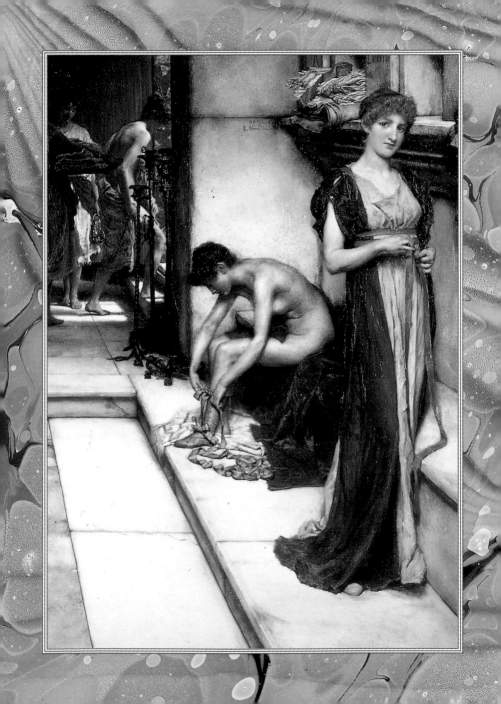

awkward position. Reflexology is based upon the belief that the soles of your feet are divided into zones that are connected to specific parts of your body: the big toe for the head; the tips of the toes for the sinuses; the base of the toes for the eyes and ears; the balls of the feet for the lungs and heart; the arch area for the stomach, kidneys, and liver; the heel for the sciatic nerve; and the ankle for the reproductive organs. Massage from the tips of the toes to the back of the ankles. Press hard and then slowly release the pressure. Be on the lookout for tender spots. These indicate areas of blocked energy. If you feel one, massage that area until the sensitivity disappears.

The Reflexology Foot Spa is healthful pampering for your body's sole support. For feets' sake, perform this fancy foot workout a couple of times a month and you'll walk through life on air.

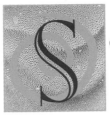

# Second Trimester Float

*I really learned it all*
*from mothers.*
— Dr. Benjamin Spock

"Congratulations, you're going to have a baby." By the sixth month you're hearing that a lot, the blessed event is starting to show, your uniform is definitely maternity, and hopefully the morning sickness is replaced by a hormone-lit glow. The Second Trimester Float is a pampering pleasure bath for expectant moms. The redolent rose-fresh fragrance is 100% ivory-pure feminine.

## The Botanicals

*Fifteen Drops of Rose Oil*
*Eight Drops of Bergamot Oil*
*Eight Drops of Rose Geranium Oil*

Joyful rose, playful bergamot, and captivating rose geranium give birth to a scent that is uplifting, refreshing, and confident. One whiff of this mood-elevating blend brings calm, soulful contentment no matter how much extra baggage is on board. The essential oils in the Second Trimester Float mother your skin with loving care. The remedial formula is toning, astringent, antiseptic, anti-inflammatory, and mildly diuretic to relieve water retention edema. The doting combination leaves your skin supple and resilient.

❈    ❈    ❈

Run your bath to a comfortable temperature, a bit cooler than usual, between 90°F and 95°F. Your natural temperature is elevated a couple of degrees during pregnancy because of the baby's body heat, so adjust the water to suit. When the tub is nearly full, add the oils of rose, bergamot, and rose geranium in that order. The impertinent scent of rose geranium intensifies the rosiness of this rich-rose aroma with sunny bergamot leading the way. Agitate the water to combine well. A floribundus fragrance fills the air.

Carefully enter the bath. For support and comfort rest your back on a bath pillow. Float and laze. Enjoy the weightless warmth. The buoyancy of the bath water displaces most of the little darling's weight to relieve the growing pressure on your back and feet. Rotate from side to side if you like, gently supporting your belly as you turn. Soak until the water cools. Pat dry and moisturize with extra care to prevent stretch marks later on. Don't be surprised if junior gifts you with a few kicks of thanks. Maybe aromatherapy works for baby, too.

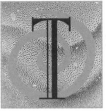ranquility Balm

*The soul is the voice*
*of the body's interests.*
— George Santayana

The Tranquility Balm is a mantra of floral essences and the ultimate bubble bath. This blessing of aromatic harmony simulates the state of higher consciousness reached during transcendental meditation. Floating for twenty minutes on a blossom-scented cloud of foam inspires exalted serenity more refreshing to body and mind than a good night's sleep.

## The Botanicals

*Two Tablespoons of Scent-Free Shampoo*

*Fifteen Drops of Neroli Oil*

*Twelve Drops of Vanilla Oil*

*Ten Drops of Carnation Oil*

The hypnotic aroma of the Tranquility Balm sustains lucid stillness and total-body relaxation. The soft-citrus scent of neroli oil, extracted from the delicate flowers of the bitter orange tree, is one of aromatherapy's most prized essences. (One ton of flowers yields one quart of oil!). Neroli's smooth, powdery aroma cultivates self-confidence, dispels anxiety, and is an antidote to depression. Diluted in bath water, its generous hydrating action benefits all skin types to facilitate cell renewal and repair tiny broken blood vessels. The warm, consoling fragrance of vanilla oil and the sweet, lightly spicy scent of carnation oil induces a glow of inner peace that strengthens the bond between happiness and healthiness to prevent illness before it starts.

❊   ❊   ❊

*To Prepare The Tranquility Bubble Bath Gel*: In a small glass bowl, combine the scent-free shampoo and the oils of neroli, vanilla, and carnation. Whisk until the mixture becomes opaque and the oils thoroughly incorporate with the scent-free shampoo. Cover the bowl and set it aside for fifteen minutes to allow the aroma to develop.

Run your bath to a pleasant temperature, between 95°F and 100°F. Pour the bubble gel into the bath, near the tap, where the water is most turbulent to make a whipped cream cloud of sweet-smelling bubbles.

Sink into the scented confection. Close your eyes and picture yourself drifting on a soft cloud covered with a warm, heaven-scented blanket of comforting bubbles. Empty your mind. It's not easy, it takes practice, but do the best you can. Try to reach the well spring of your spirit, the psychic source of your inner strength. The beautiful fragrance is your transportation to this blissful state of tranquility.

# 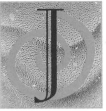asmine Beta Boost

*Something deeply hidden
had to be behind things.*
— Albert Einstein

Count on an American sneaker company to be at the cutting edge of aromatherapy research. At the Taste and Scent Treatment Center in Chicago, Nike made a surprising discovery: The demure scent of jasmine oil packs a powerful psychic punch. Extracted from the star-shaped petals of the tiny, night-blooming flower, *eau de jasmin* fires a storm of beta waves that activates the brain to be super alert and productive. Combine a dash of uplifting oil of geranium and a twist of lively oil of lemon with the mostly-jasmine blend to excite an *après le bain* brainstorm of vital energy.

## The Botanicals

*Five Drops of Geranium Oil
Eight Drops of Lemon Oil
Twenty Drops of Jasmine Oil*

The Jasmine Beta Boost is a bath with a practical purpose. A fifteen to twenty minute soak, inhaling the rich mixture of power odors, fortifies mental agility and makes your mind sharp as a tack. The two mood-elevating top notes, oil of geranium and oil of lemon, sparkle in tandem to deepen the delicate, powdery scent of jasmine, the Beta Boost's bottom note. Deep breaths of spicy-clean geranium oil relieves stress and buttresses self-confidence. Sassy and citrus-sweet, oil of lemon acts on your senses just the way it smells: refreshing, uplifting, and rejuvenating. The delicate, lingering fragrance of the wonder-flower jasmine sparks flashes of insight to keep you keen-witted and brainy.

✿   ✿   ✿

Run your bath to a comfortable temperature, between 95°F and 100°F. When the tub is almost full, add the geranium oil, the lemon oil, and the oil of jasmine. Deliver the oils into the bathwater in the prescribed order. The soft, floral scent of jasmine oil is added last to ensure its dominance over the penetrating scent of geranium. Between applications, clean the glass dropper to avoid contaminating your bottles of essential oil. Gently disturb the bath water with your hand to disperse and combine all of the ingredients evenly.

Slip into the steaming water. As the aroma envelops you, let go of negative emotions: anger, guilt, free-floating anxiety. The arousing fragrance of the Jasmine Beta Boost is a psychic weapon against the clever bully, Stress. Inhale deeply. Let the layers of heady scent reinforce your natural sense of self-confidence and courage. You know you're the best, now you're ready to go out and prove it.

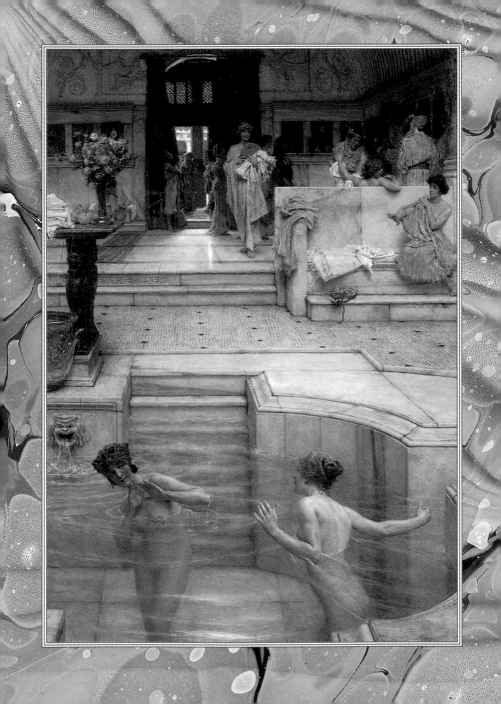

# AROMATHERAPY Home-Shopping Network

Aphrodisia
264 Bleecker Street
New York, NY 10014
(212) 989-6440
*Dried herbs, essential oils*

Aroma Vera Inc.
P.O. Box 3609
Culver City, CA 90231
(310) 280-0407
*Bath & skincare products, essential oils*

Bare Escentuals
1300 Industrial Road, Ste. #14
San Carlos, CA 94070
(800) 227-3990
*Bath & skincare products, essential oils*

The Body Shop By Mail
45 Horsehill Road
Hanover Technical Center
Cedar Knolls, NJ 07927
(800) 541-2535
*Bath & skincare products, essential oils*

Body Time
1341 Seventh Street
Berkeley, CA 94710
(510) 524-0360
*Aromatherapy, bath & skincare products,
essential oils*

Capriland's Herb Farm
Silver Street
North Coventry, CT 06238
(203) 742-7244
*Dried herbs, essential oils*

Caswell-Massey Catalog
Catalog Division
100 Enterprise Place
Dover, DE 19901
(800) 326-0500
*Bath & skincare products, essential oils*

Common Scents Catalog
3920 24th Street
San Francisco, CA 94114
(415) 826-1019
*Bath & skincare products, essential oils*

Crabtree & Evelyn Catalog
Mail Order Division
P.O. Box 158
Woodstock, CT 06281
(800) 272-2873
*Bath & skincare products, essential oils*
*[essential oils not in mail order catalog]*

Culpeper Ltd.
21 Bruton Street
London W1X 7DA, England
44-171-499-2406
*Dried herbs, essential oils*

Czech & Speake Catalog
39C Jermyn Street
London SW1 6JH, England
44-171-439-0216
*Bath & skincare products, essential oils*

D. Napier & Sons
17 Bristol Place
Edinburgh, EHI, Scotland
44-131-225-5542
*Dried herbs*

Devonshire Apothecary
P.O. Box 160215
Austin, TX 78716-0215
(512) 477-8270
*Aromatherapy, bath & skincare products,
dried herbs*

Energy Essentials
P.O. Box 470785
San Francisco, CA 94147
(415) 753-3382
*Essential oils*

Essentially Yours
P.O. Box 38
Romford, Essex RM1 DN
England
*Essential oils*

Farmaceutica di Santa Maria Novella
Via della Scala, 16
50123, Florence, Italy
39-55-216276
*Bath & skincare products, essential oils*

Frontier Cooperative Herbs
Box 299
Norway, IA 52318
(800) 786-1388
*Bath & skincare products, dried herbs [organic],
essential oils*

Gaia Products
62 Kent Street
Brooklyn, NY 11222
(718) 389-8224
*Dried herbs, essential oils*

Green Mountain Herbs Ltd.
P.O. Box 2369
Boulder, CO 80306
(800) 525-2696
*Dried herbs, essential oils*

Hausmann's Pharmacy, Inc.
534-536 W. Girard Avenue
Philadelphia, PA 19123
(800) 235-5522
*Dried herbs, essential oils*

Hove Parfumeur Ltd. Catalog
824 Royal Street
New Orleans, LA 70116
(504) 525-7827
*Essential oils*

John Bell & Croyden
Department A6MO
52-54 Wigmore Street
London, W.I. England
44-171-935-5555
*Essential oils*

Kiehl's Pharmacy
109 Third Avenue
New York, NY 10003
(212) 475-3400
*Skincare products, essential oils*

Nature's Herb
1010 46th Street
Emeryville, CA 94608
(510) 601-0700
*Dried herbs, essential oils*

Original Swiss Aromatics
Pacific Institute of Aromatherapy
P.O. Box 6842
San Rafael, CA 94903
(415) 459-3998
*Aromatherapy supplies, essential oils*

SelfCare Catalog
5850 Shellmound Street
Emeryville, CA 94608
(800) 345-3371
*Aromatherapy, bath & skincare products*

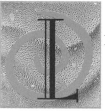

# ist Of Illustrations

*Grateful acknowledgment is made for
permission to reproduce the following works of
art by Sir Lawrence Alma-Tadema:*

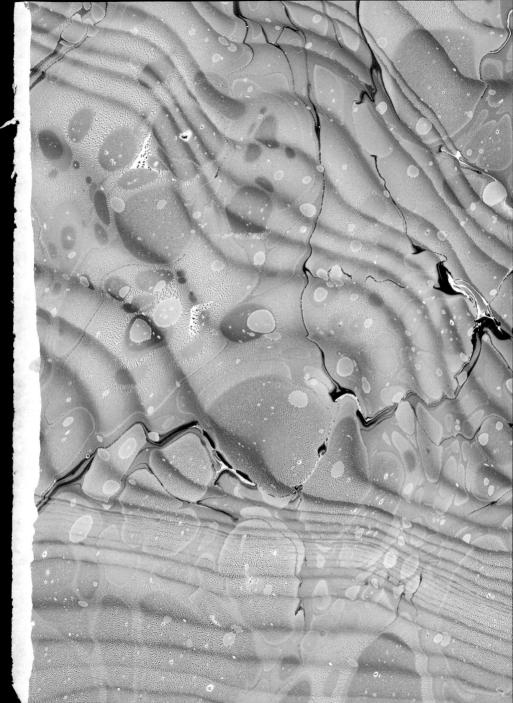

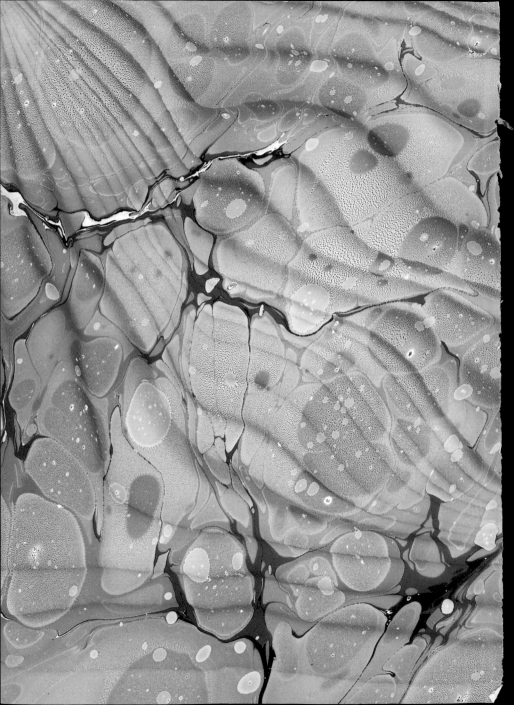